TYPE 1

DIABETES

COOKBOOK

For Kids

Delicious Low Carb Recipes
Every Child Would Want To Eat

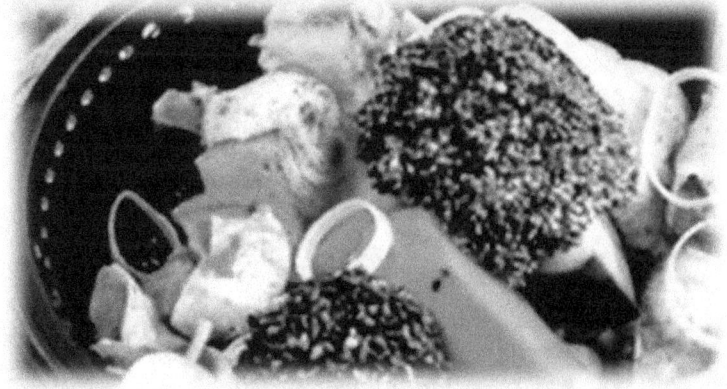

Dr. Grace Hester A.kaboo Publishing —

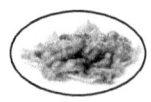 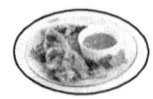 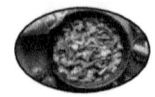

Copyright Page

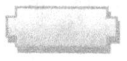

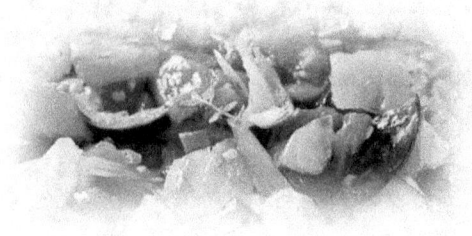

Disclaimer: The recipes contained in this cookbook are intended for personal use and enjoyment. The author and publisher are not responsible for any health issues or allergic reactions that may arise from the use of the ingredients or recipes provided. It is recommended that individuals with specific dietary concerns or restrictions consult a qualified healthcare professional.

DR.GRACE
HESTER

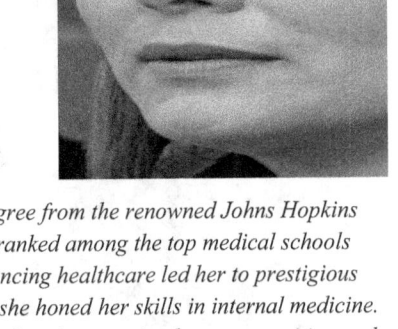

.Dr. Grace Hester stands at the intersection of health, passion, and culinary excellence. A distinguished medical professional and accomplished nutritionist, she seamlessly weaves together her expertise to create a holistic approach to well-being.

Dr. Hester earned her medical degree from the renowned Johns Hopkins School of Medicine, consistently ranked among the top medical schools globally. Her commitment to advancing healthcare led her to prestigious positions at the Mayo Clinic, where she honed her skills in internal medicine. Driven by a desire to explore the profound connection between nutrition and overall health, she furthered her education at the Culinary Institute of America.

– With a deep understanding of both medicine and nutrition, Dr. Hester embarked on a mission to inspire others to embrace a healthier lifestyle. Her culinary journey– led to the creation of a series of cookbooks that blend the art of cooking with the science of nutrition. Each recipe is a testament to her commitment to flavor, nourishment, and well-being.–

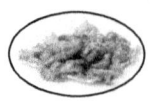 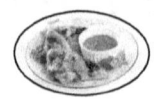 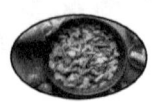

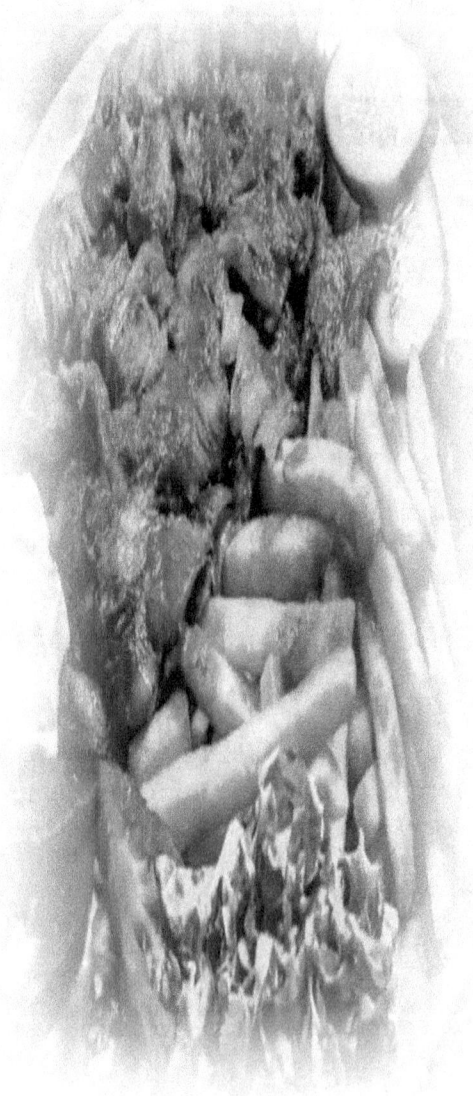

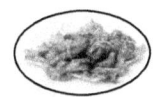 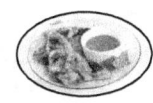 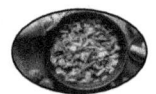

TABLE OF CONTENT

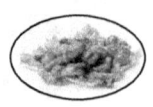 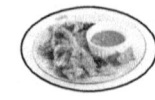 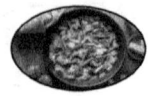

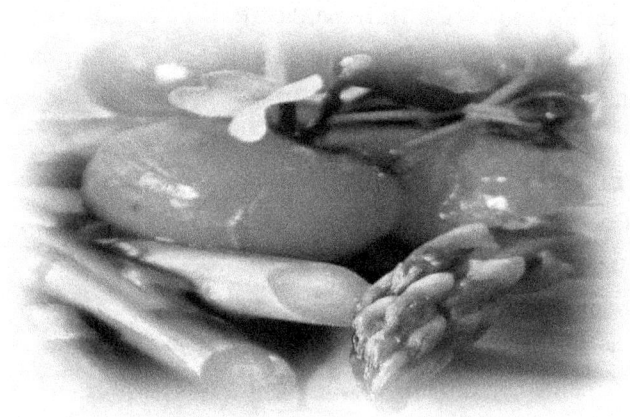

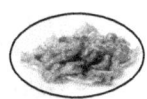 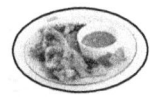 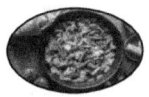

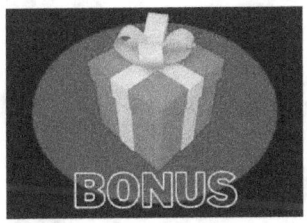

SCAN THE QR CODE TO GET YOUR FREE HOME
MADE GREEN SMOOTHIE RECIPE BOOK

Your 20 days meal planner is attached at the end of the
book. Enjoy!

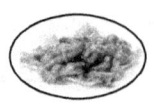 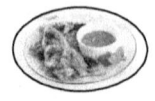 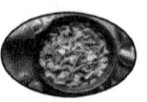

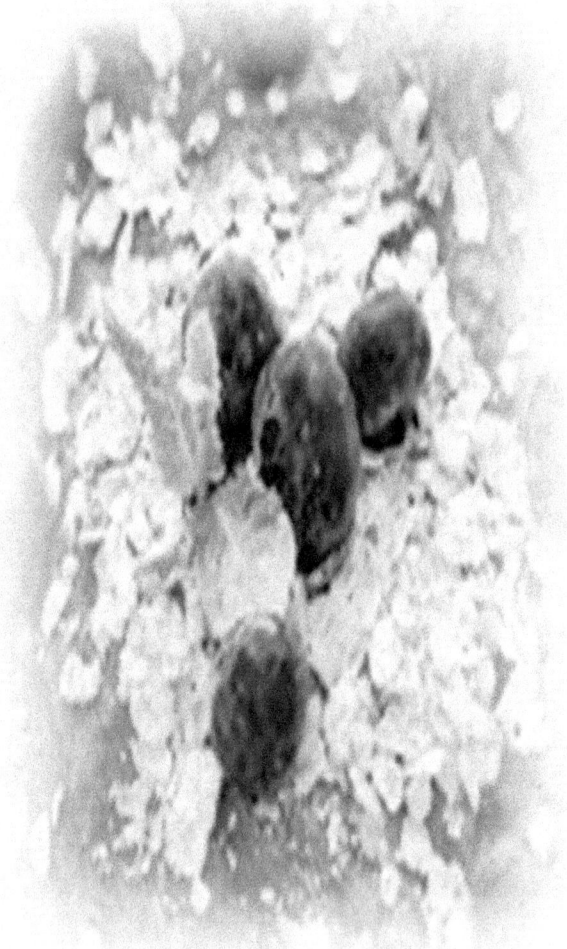

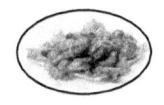 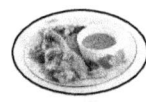 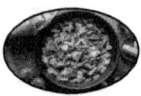

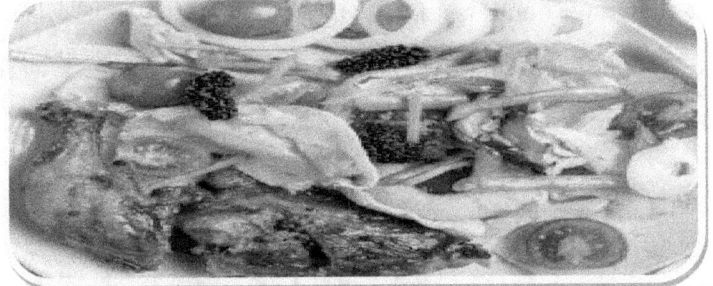

INTRODUCTION-

"CARB CRUNCHERS: A TYPE 1 DIABETES COOKBOOK FOR KIDS"

Meet Oliver, an adventurous 10-year-old with a love for exploration and a spirit as boundless as the sky. Oliver, however, faced a unique challenge—Type 1 diabetes. Navigating the world of carb counting, insulin shots, and blood sugar checks wasn't always easy, especially for a young explorer with a penchant for excitement.

One day, Oliver's mom stumbled upon a treasure trove—the "Carb Crunchers" cookbook specially crafted for kids like him. This culinary guide promised not just low-carb meals –

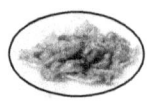 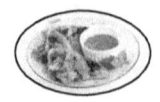 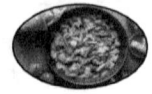

but delicious delights that would make every child's taste buds dance. Little did Oliver know that these recipes were about to transform his world.

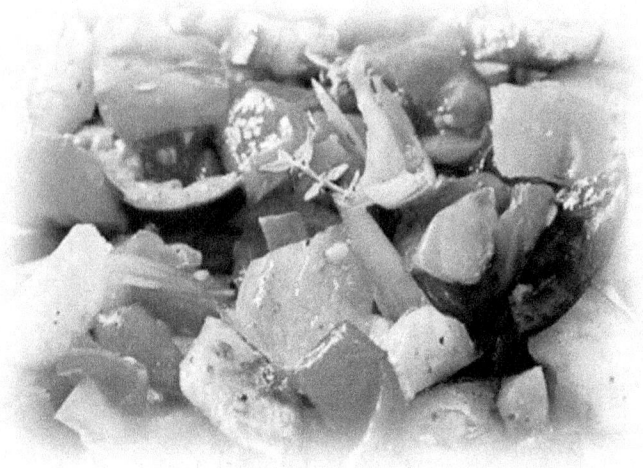

As Oliver dove into the cookbook, he discovered a universe of mouthwatering possibilities. Gone were the days of feeling limited by dietary restrictions. Instead, he found himself crafting Pizza Zucchini Boats that sailed into the realm of flavor, and Chicken and Broccoli Casserole that was a symphony of textures and tastes.–

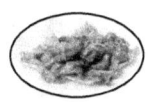 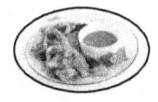 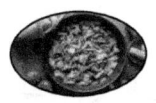

But it wasn't just about meals; "Carb Crunchers" became Oliver's kitchen companion, helping him concoct Turkey and Veggie Roll-Ups for school lunches and surprising his taste buds with the Cauliflower Mac 'n' Cheese that felt like a secret indulgence.

Each recipe was like a chapter in Oliver's culinary adventure, from the vibrant Berry Parfait that added a burst of color to his mornings to the Veggie Egg Muffins that made breakfast an exciting affair. His friends, once skeptical of "diabetic food," soon found themselves joining in the feast, realizing that low-carb could be synonymous with high flavor.

Oliver's lunchbox, once a source of hesitation, became a treasure trove of goodness with Peanut Butter Banana Smoothies and Turkey and Cheese Quesadillas stealing the show. Avocado Chicken Salad, with its creamy goodness, became the envy of the school cafeteria.

As the days passed, Oliver's energy levels soared, his blood sugar levels stabilized, and his zest for life grew stronger. "Carb Crunchers" had turned his kitchen into a magical realm where every dish was a triumph and a celebration.–

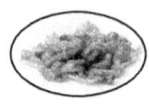 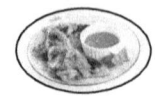 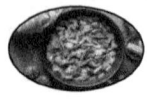

This cookbook didn't just change Oliver's diet; it transformed his perspective on living with Type 1 diabetes. It became a tale of resilience, creativity, and, most importantly, delicious victories. Now, as Oliver embarks on each new day, he carries the wisdom of "Carb Crunchers" and the flavors of a life not just managed but savored.

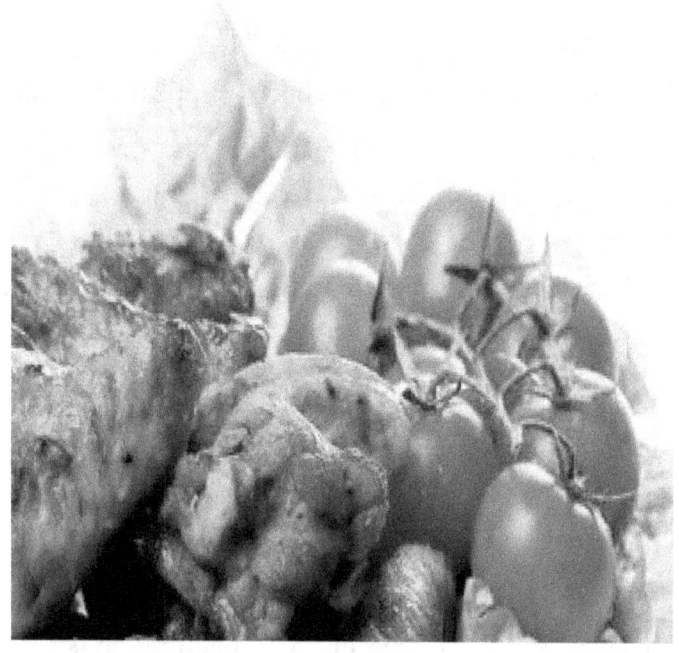

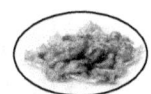 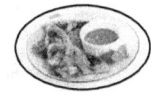 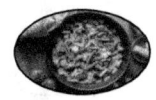

Ingredients:

- 4 medium zucchinis

- 1 cup sugar-free marinara sauce

- 1 cup shredded mozzarella cheese

- 1/2 cu p mini pepperoni slices

- 1 tsp Italian seasoning

- Salt and pepper to taste

—

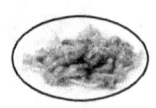 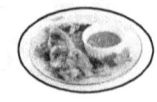 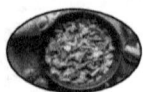

Instructions:

1. Preheat the oven to 400°F (200°C).

2. Cut each zucchini in half lengthwise and scoop out the seeds to create a "boat."

3. The zucchinis should be placed on a baking sheet.

4. Spread marinara sauce evenly on each zucchini boat.

5. Sprinkle mozzarella cheese over the sauce.

6. Add mini pepperoni slices on top.

7. Sprinkle with Italian seasoning, salt, and pepper.

8. Baking should be done for about 20 minutes

9. Let it cool slightly before serving.

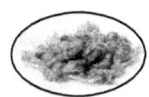 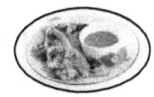 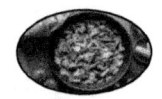

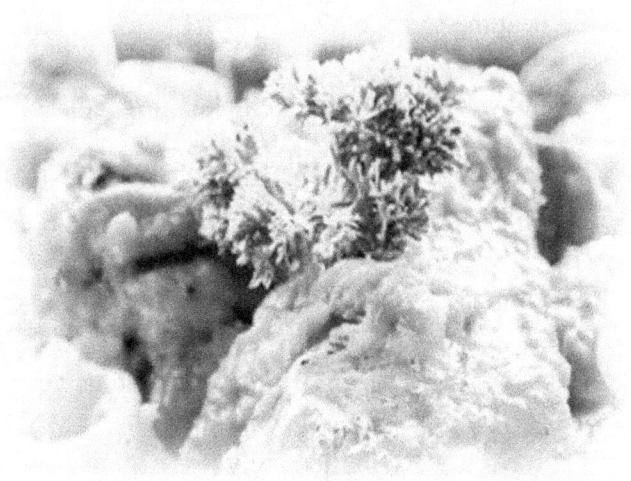

Ingredients:

- 2 cups cooked chicken, shredded

- 2 cups broccoli florets

- 1 cup cheddar cheese, shredded

- 1/2 cup mayonnaise

- 1/2 cup sour cream

- 1 tsp garlic powder

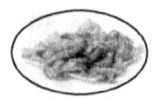 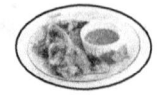 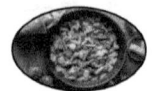

- Salt and pepper to taste

Instructions:

1. Preheat the oven to 375°F (190°C).

2. In a bowl, mix shredded chicken, broccoli, cheddar cheese, mayonnaise, sour cream, garlic powder, salt, and pepper.

3. The mixture should be send to a baking dish.

4. Bake for 25-30 minutes or until golden and bubbly.

5. Proceed to serve immediately it is cooled..

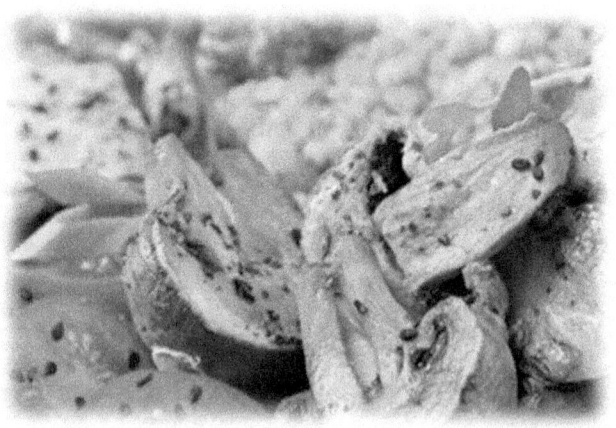

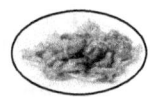 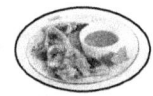 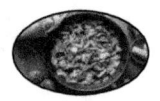

3. TURKEY AND VEGGIE ROLL-UPS

Ingredients:

- 8 slices turkey or chicken breast

- 1/2 cup cream cheese

- 1/4 cup diced bell peppers

- 1/4 cup shredded carrots

- 1/4 cup cucumber, thinly sliced

- Salt and pepper to taste

Instructions:

1. Lay out turkey slices on a flat surface.

2. In a bowl, mix cream cheese, bell peppers, shredded carrots, salt, and pepper.

3. Spread the cream cheese mixture on each turkey slice.

4. Place a few cucumber slices on one end of each slice.

5. Roll up the turkey slices and secure with toothpicks.

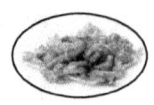 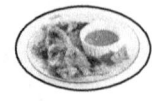 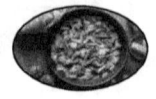

6. Refrigerate for 30 minutes before slicing into bite-sized pieces.

Ingredients:

- one average cauliflower head, ensure you cut into florets

- 1 cup cheddar cheese, shredded

- 1/2 cup heavy cream

- 2 tbsp unsalted butter

- 1 tsp mustard powder

- Salt and pepper to taste

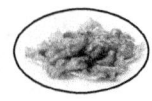 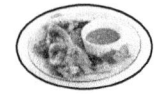 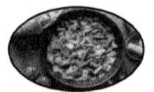

Instructions:

1. Steam cauliflower until tender.

2. In a saucepan, melt butter and add heavy cream, mustard powder, salt, and pepper.

3. Stir in cheddar cheese until smooth.

4. Mix the cheese sauce with the steamed cauliflower.

5. Bake at 350°F (175°C) for 15-20 minutes or until golden.

5. BERRY PARFAIT

Ingredients:

- one cup of mixed or different berries such as strawberries, blueberries, raspberries etc

- 1 cup Greek yogurt

- 1/4 cup almond slices

- 1 tbsp honey (optional)

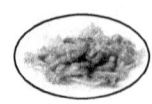 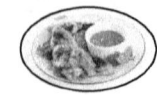 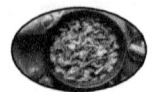

Instructions:

1. In a glass, layer mixed berries and Greek yogurt.

2. until the glass is filled continually repeat the layers

3. Top with almond slices and drizzle with honey if desired.

6. VEGGIE EGG MUFFINS

Ingredients:

- 6 eggs

- 1/2 cup bell peppers, diced

- 1/2 cup spinach, chopped

- 1/4 cup feta cheese, crumbled

- Salt and pepper to taste

—

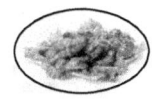 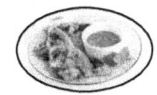 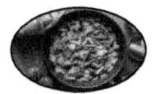

Instructions:

1. Preheat the oven to 350°F (175°C).

2. In a bowl, beat the eggs and add diced bell peppers, chopped spinach, feta cheese, salt, and pepper.

3. Pour the mixture into greased muffin cups.

4. Bake for 20-25 minutes or until the eggs are set.

7. PEANUT BUTTER BANANA SMOOTHIE

Ingredients:

- 1 ripe banana

- 2 tbsp peanut butter

- 1 cup unsweetened almond milk

- Ice cubes

Instructions:

1. Blend banana, peanut butter, almond milk, and ice cubes until smooth.

2. Pour into a glass and serve immediately.

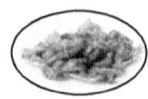 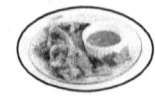 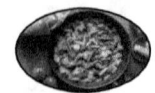

8. TURKEY AND CHEESE QUESADILLAS

Ingredients:

- 4 low-carb tortillas

- 1 cup turkey slices

- 1 cup cheddar cheese, shredded

- 1/4 cup salsa (optional)

- Cooking spray

Instructions:

1. Place a tortilla on a flat surface and add turkey slices and cheddar cheese.

2. Top with another tortilla.

3. Heat a skillet over medium heat and coat with cooking spray.

4. Cook the quesadilla for 2-3 minutes on each side until cheese melts.

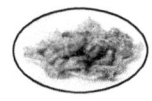 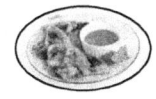 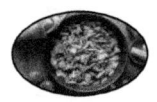

5. Cut into wedges and serve with salsa if desired.

9. AVOCADO CHICKEN SALAD

Ingredients:

- 2 cups cooked chicken, shredded

- 1 avocado, diced

- 1/4 cup red onion, finely chopped

- 1/4 cup mayonnaise

- 1 tbsp lime juice

- Salt and pepper to taste

Instructions:

1. In a bowl, mix shredded chicken, diced avocado, red onion, mayonnaise, lime juice, salt, and pepper.

2. Stir until well combined.

3. Chill in the refrigerator before serving.

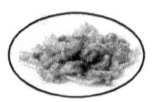 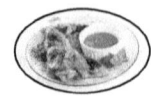 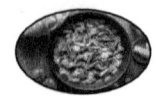

Ingredients:

- 4 boneless, skinless chicken breasts

- 2 cups broccoli florets, steamed

- 1 cup cheddar cheese, shredded

- 1 tsp garlic powder

- Salt and pepper to taste

Instructions:

1. Preheat the oven to 375°F (190°C).

2. . Use salt, pepper, and garlic powder to season chicken breasts.

3. . Slit each chicken breast into a pocket.

4. . Stuff cheddar cheese and cooked broccoli into each pocket.–

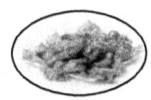 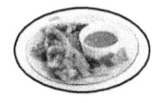 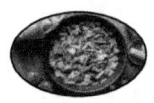

5. . Bake the chicken for 25 to 30 minutes, or until it is thoroughly done.

11. CHEESY SPINACH STUFFED MUSHROOMS

Ingredients:

- Twelve big mushrooms, cleaned, de-stemmed

- 1 cup spinach, chopped

- 1/2 cup cream cheese

- 1/4 cup Parmesan cheese, grated

- 2 cloves garlic, minced

- Salt and pepper to taste

Instructions:

1. Preheat the oven to 375°F (190°C).

2. In a pan, sauté chopped spinach and minced garlic until wilted.–

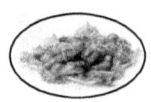 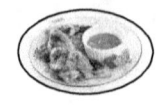 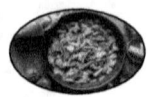

3. In a bowl, mix the sautéed spinach with cream cheese, Parmesan cheese, salt, and pepper.

4. Fill each mushroom cap with the spinach and cheese mixture.

5. Bake for 15-20 minutes or until mushrooms are tender.

12. GRILLED CHICKEN SKEWERS WITH DIPPING SAUCE

Ingredients:

- Two skinless, boneless chicken breasts that have been cubed

- 1 bell pepper, cut into chunks

- 1 zucchini, sliced

- 1/4 cup olive oil

- 1 tsp paprika

- 1/2 tsp cumin

- Salt and pepper to taste

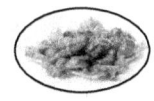 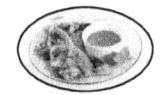 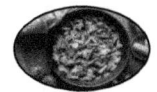

Instructions:

1. Preheat the grill or grill pan.

2. In a bowl, mix chicken cubes, bell pepper chunks, and zucchini slices with olive oil, paprika, cumin, salt, and pepper.

3. Thread the chicken and veggies onto skewers.

4. Grill for 8-10 minutes, turning occasionally, until chicken is cooked through.

5. Serve with a side of low-carb dipping sauce.

13. MINI CAPRESE SALAD SKEWERS

Ingredients:

- 12 cherry tomatoes

- 12 mini mozzarella balls

- Fresh basil leaves

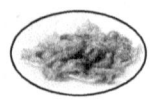 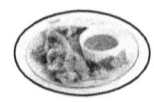 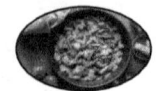

- Balsamic glaze for drizzling

- Salt and pepper to taste

Instructions:

1. Thread a tomato, a mozzarella ball, and a basil leaf onto small skewers.

2. Arrange the skewers on a serving platter.

3. After adding a balsamic glaze, season with salt and pepper.

14. TUNA LETTUCE WRAPS

Ingredients:

- 1 can tuna, drained

- 1/4 cup mayonnaise

- 1 celery stalk, finely chopped

- 1 tbsp Dijon mustard

- Lettuce leaves for wrapping–

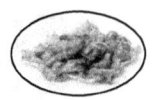 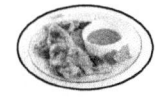 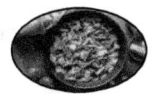

Instructions:

1. In a bowl, mix tuna, mayonnaise, chopped celery, and Dijon mustard.

2. Spoon the tuna mixture onto lettuce leaves.

3. Wrap and secure with toothpicks for a tasty and low-carb alternative.

15. Chocolate Avocado Pudding

Ingredients:

- 2 ripe avocados

- 1/4 cup unsweetened cocoa powder

- 1/4 cup almond milk

- 2 tbsp low-carb sweetener

- 1 tsp vanilla extract

—

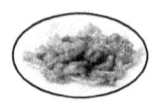 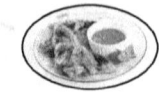 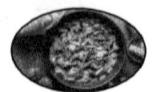

Instructions:

1. In a blender, combine avocados, cocoa powder, almond milk, sweetener, and vanilla extract.

2. Blend until smooth and creamy.

3. Put in refrigerator for at least 58 minutes before serving.

16. Asian Chicken Lettuce Wraps

Ingredients:

- 1 lb ground chicken

- 1/4 cup soy sauce

- 2 tbsp hoisin sauce

- 1 tbsp sesame oil

- 2 green onions, sliced

- 1/4 cup water chestnuts, chopped

- Lettuce leaves for wrapping

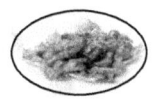 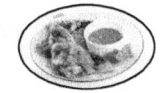 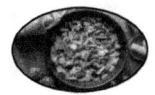

Instructions:

1. In a skillet, cook ground chicken until browned.

2. Stir in soy sauce, hoisin sauce, sesame oil, green onions, and water chestnuts.

3. Simmer for 5-7 minutes.

4. Spoon the chicken mixture onto lettuce leaves and wrap.

17. CUCUMBER AND CREAM CHEESE SANDWICHES

Ingredients:

- 1 cucumber, thinly sliced

- 8 oz cream cheese, softened

- Fresh dill, chopped

- Salt and pepper to taste

- Low-carb bread or cucumber slices for serving–

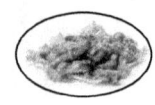 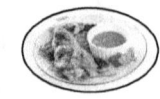 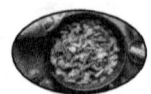

Instructions:

1. In a bowl, mix cream cheese, chopped dill, salt, and pepper.

2. Spread the cream cheese mixture on low-carb bread or cucumber slices.

3. Top with thinly sliced cucumber.

18. EGG SALAD LETTUCE WRAPS

Ingredients:

- 6 hard-boiled eggs, chopped

- 1/4 cup mayonnaise

- 1 tsp Dijon mustard

- 2 tbsp chives, chopped

- Lettuce leaves for wrapping

—

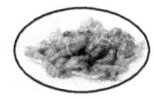 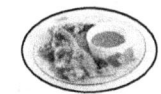 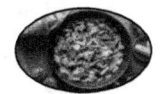

Instructions:

1. In a bowl, combine chopped hard-boiled eggs, mayonnaise, Dijon mustard, and chopped chives.

2. Spoon the egg salad onto lettuce leaves and wrap for a delicious and carb-friendly lunch.

19. ZESTY SHRIMP SKEWERS

Ingredients:

- 1 lb shrimp, peeled and deveined

- 2 tbsp olive oil

- 1 tsp paprika

- 1/2 tsp garlic powder

- Zest and juice of one lemon

- Salt and pepper to taste

—

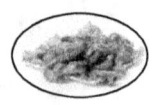 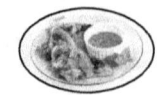 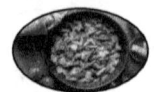

Instructions:

1. In a bowl, toss shrimp with olive oil, paprika, garlic powder, lemon zest, lemon juice, salt, and pepper.

2. Thread the shrimp onto skewers.

3. Grill for 2-3 minutes per side until shrimp are opaque and cooked through.

20. Veggie and Cheese Stuffed Bell Peppers

Ingredients:

- 4 bell peppers, halved and seeds removed

- 1 cup cauliflower rice

- 1/2 cup shredded cheddar cheese

- 1/4 cup salsa (optional)

- 1 tsp cumin

- Salt and pepper to taste

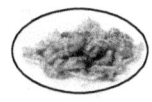 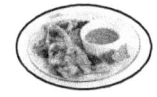 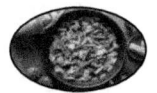

Instructions:

1. Preheat the oven to 375°F (190°C).

2. In a bowl, mix cauliflower rice, cheddar cheese, salsa (if using), cumin, salt, and pepper.

3. Stuff each bell pepper half with the veggie and cheese mixture.

4. Baking should be done for 25minuts or thirty minutes

Ingredients:

- 1 cup cherry tomatoes

- 1 cup cucumber, diced

- 1 cup feta cheese, cubed

- Kalamata olives (optional)

- Olive oil and oregano for drizzling

- Salt and pepper to taste–

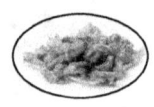 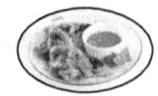 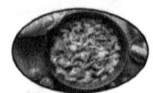

Instructions:

1. Thread cherry tomatoes, cucumber, and feta cheese alternately onto small skewers.

2. Add Kalamata olives if desired.

3. Drizzle with olive oil, sprinkle with oregano, salt, and pepper.

22. SPINACH AND FETA STUFFED CHICKEN BREAST

Ingredients:

- 4 boneless, skinless chicken breasts

- 2 cups fresh spinach, chopped

- 1/2 cup feta cheese, crumbled

- 2 cloves garlic, minced

- 1 tbsp olive oil

- Salt and pepper to taste

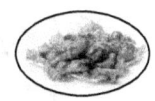 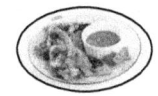 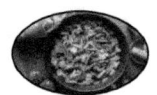

Instructions:

1. Preheat the oven to 375°F (190°C).

2. In a skillet, sauté chopped spinach and minced garlic in olive oil until wilted.

3. Slice a pocket into each chicken breast.

4. Stuff each pocket with the sautéed spinach and crumbled feta.

5. Season with salt and pepper.

6. Bake for 25-30 minutes or until chicken is cooked through.

23. TURKEY AND VEGGIE MEATBALLS

Ingredients:

- 1 lb ground turkey

- 1/2 cup zucchini, grated

- 1/2 cup carrot, grated

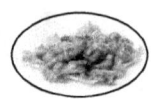 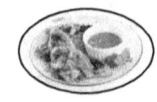 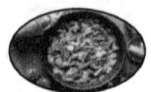

- 1/4 cup almond flour

- 1 egg

- 1 tsp Italian seasoning

- Salt and pepper to taste

Instructions:

1. Preheat the oven to 375°F (190°C).

2. In a bowl, combine ground turkey, grated zucchini, grated carrot, almond flour, egg, Italian seasoning, salt, and pepper.

3. Place the meatballs on a baking sheet after shaping the ingredients into them.

4. Bake till cooked through, 20 to 25 minutes.

—

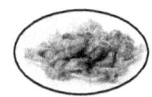 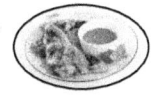 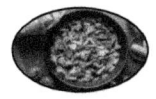

Ingredients:

- 2 cups almond flour

- 1/4 cup coconut flour

- 1/2 cup low-carb sweetener

- 1 tsp baking powder

- 1/2 cup butter, melted

- 4 large eggs

- 1 tsp vanilla extract

- 1 cup mixed berries (blueberries, raspberries)

Instructions:

1. Preheat the oven to 350°F (175°C).

2. In a bowl, mix almond flour, coconut flour, sweetener, and baking powder

3. Combine the eggs, vanilla extract, and melted butter in another bowl.

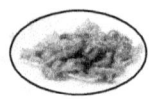 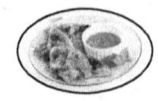 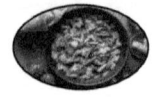

4. . Mix the dry and wet ingredients together, then gently fold in the mixed berries.

5. . Fill muffin tins with batter, bake for 20 to 25 minutes. King powder.

25. CAULIFLOWER TOTS

Ingredients:

- 2 cups cauliflower rice

- 1 cup sharp cheddar cheese, shredded

- 1/4 cup almond flour

- 1/4 cup Parmesan cheese, grated

- 1 egg

- 1 tsp garlic powder

- Salt and pepper to taste

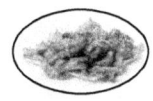 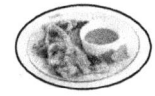 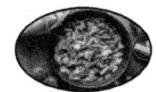

Instructions:

1. Preheat the oven to 400°F (200°C).

2. In a bowl, mix cauliflower rice, cheddar cheese, almond flour, Parmesan cheese, egg, garlic powder, salt, and pepper.

3. Form the mixture into tot shapes and place on a baking sheet.

4. Baking should be done for at least 20-25 minutes

26. SOUTHWEST STUFFED PEPPERS

Ingredients:

- 4 bell peppers, halved and seeds removed

- 1 lb ground beef or turkey

- 1 cup cauliflower rice

- 1/2 cup black beans, drained and rinsed

- 1/2 cup salsa

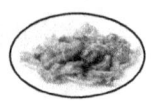 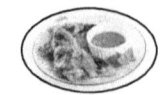 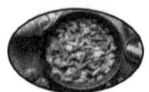

- 1 tsp cumin

- 1/2 tsp chili powder

- Salt and pepper to taste

- Shredded cheddar cheese for topping

Instructions:

1. Preheat the oven to 375°F (190°C).

2. Brown ground beef or turkey in a skillet.

3. In a bowl, mix cooked meat, cauliflower rice, black beans, salsa, cumin, chili powder, salt, and pepper.

4. Stuff each bell pepper half with the mixture.

5. Top with shredded cheddar cheese.

6. Baking should be done for at least 25-30 minutes.–

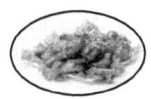 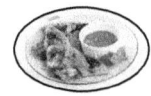 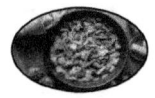

Ingredients:

- 4 cups fresh spinach

- 1 cup strawberries, sliced

- 1/4 cup feta cheese, crumbled

- 1/4 cup almonds, sliced

- Balsamic vinaigrette dressing

Instructions:

1. In a large bowl, combine fresh spinach, sliced strawberries, crumbled feta, and sliced almonds.

2. Toss gently to coat after drizzling with balsamic vinaigrette dressing.

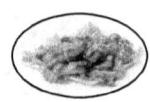 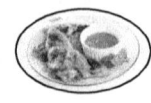 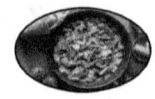

Ingredients:

- 1 lb ground turkey

- 1/2 cup bell peppers, diced

- 1/2 cup water chestnuts, chopped

- 1/4 cup soy sauce

- 1 tsp ginger, minced

- Lettuce leaves for wrapping

Instructions:

1. In a skillet, cook ground turkey until browned.

2. Add diced bell peppers, water chestnuts, soy sauce, and minced ginger.

3. Cook for an additional 5-7 minutes.

4. Spoon the turkey mixture onto lettuce leaves and wrap.–

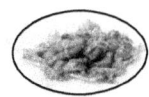 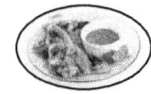 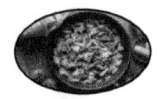

Ingredients:

- 1 cup almond butter

- 1/2 cup almond flour

- 1/4 cup low-carb sweetener

- 1 tsp vanilla extract

- 1/2 cup dark chocolate chips

- 1/4 cup shredded coconut (optional)

Instructions:

1. In a bowl, mix almond butter, almond flour, sweetener, and vanilla extract.

2. Fold in dark chocolate chips.

3. Roll the mixture into bite-sized balls.

4. Optionally, roll each ball in shredded coconut.–

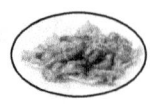 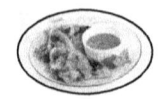 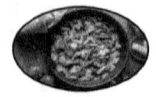

5. Let it cool for a minimum of half an hour before serving.

30. Caprese Stuffed Avocados

Ingredients:

- 4 ripe avocados

- 1 cup cherry tomatoes, halved

- 1 cup fresh mozzarella balls

- Fresh basil leaves, chopped

- Balsamic glaze for drizzling

- Salt and pepper to taste

Instructions:

1. . Halve the avocados and remove the pits.

2. In a bowl, mix cherry tomatoes, fresh mozzarella, chopped basil, salt, and pepper.

3. Spoon the caprese mixture into each avocado half.

4. Drizzle with balsamic glaze before serving.

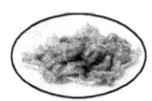 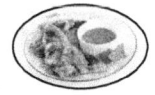 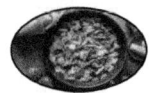

CONCLUSION

A Culinary Adventure Unveiled

As we close the pages of "Carb Crunchers: A Type 1 Diabetes Cookbook for Kids," we find ourselves in the heartwarming aftermath of a culinary journey—a journey that transcended the limitations of a health condition and transformed them into opportunities for creativity, joy, and delicious discovery.

Oliver's story serves as an inspiration, a testament to the power of thoughtful, nutritious, and tasty recipes in the lives of children with Type 1 diabetes. With each recipe, we witnessed not just a change in his diet but a profound shift in his outlook. The once-daunting prospect of managing blood sugar levels became an adventure in the kitchen, filled with laughter, experimentation, and newfound confidence.

"Carb Crunchers" isn't merely a cookbook; it's a guide to reimagining meals, a companion on the journey to health, and a source of empowerment for both kids and parents alike. From the delightful Pizza Zucchini Boats to the

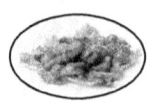 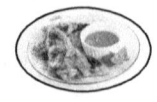 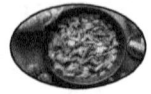

comforting Cauliflower Mac 'n' Cheese, these recipes are bridges to a world where flavor isn't sacrificed for health—it's celebrated.

In the end, this book is a celebration of resilience, a reminder that life's challenges can be met with creativity and joy. As the aroma of Turkey and Veggie Roll-Ups fills the kitchen and the laughter of children enjoying Chocolate Avocado Pudding echoes in the air, we see the impact of small changes—changes that ripple through lives, transforming meals into moments of triumph and shared happiness.

To every child, parent, and caregiver embracing the journey of managing Type 1 diabetes, may "Carb Crunchers" be a source of inspiration, a trusted ally in the kitchen, and a reminder that every meal is an opportunity to savor life's flavors to the fullest. As Oliver's tale concludes, a new chapter begins for each reader—filled with the promise of delicious possibilities, one recipe at a time.

Happy cooking, happy eating, and here's to a future where every bite is a step towards health, happiness, and a life well-lived.

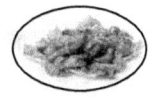 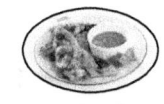 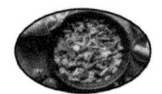

THANK YOU...

THAT'S WHY WE ARE SAYING THANK YOU...

"We know time is the unit of destiny, that's why we are saying thank you."

Dear Valued Customer,

we understand that time is a precious commodity, and we sincerely appreciate you choosing to spend a portion of it with us. Your decision to trust us with your purchase means the world to us, and we want to express our deepest gratitude.

Your support not only fuels our passion for delivering quality products but also contributes to the destiny of our business. Each customer is a vital part of our journey, and we are honored to have you

We strive to provide an exceptional shopping experience, and your satisfaction is our top priority. If you have any feedback or suggestions, we would love to hear from you. Your insights help us improve.

As a small token of our appreciation, we kindly invite you to share your experience by leaving a 5-star review. Your feedback not only boosts our morale but also assists fellow shoppers in making informed decisions.

Once again, thank you for choosing to buy this book. We look forward to serving you again and being a part of your destiny in the world of quality and excellence.

Warm regards,

Dr. Grace Hester–

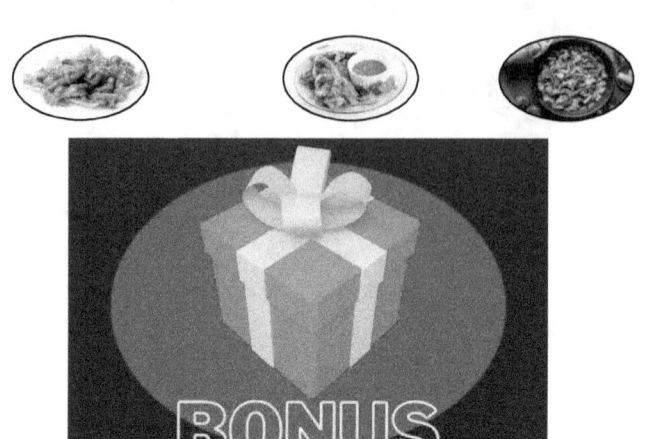

20 DAYS + MEAL PLANNER

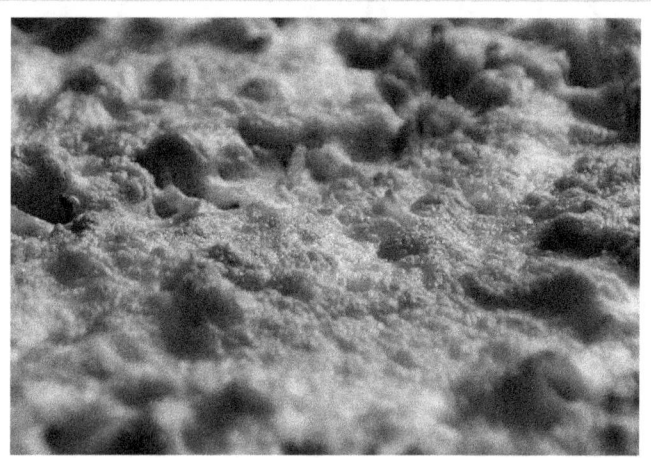

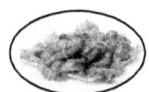
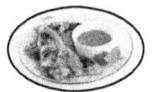
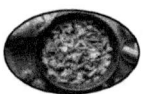

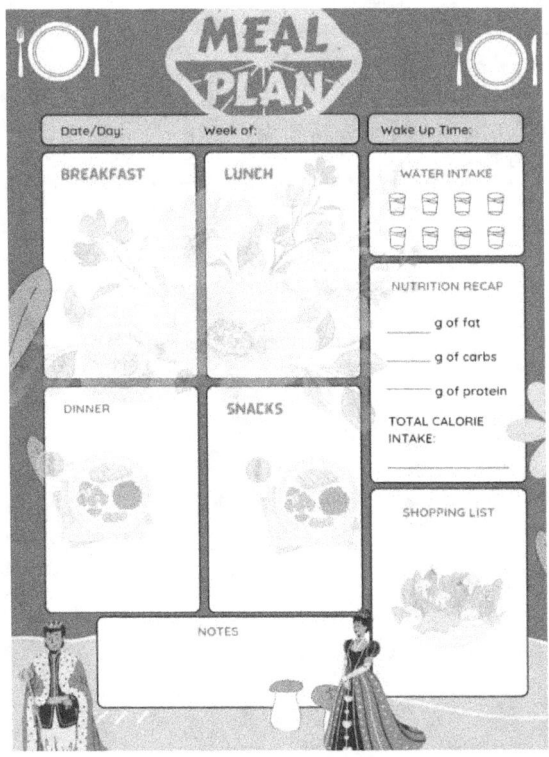

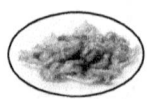
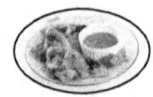
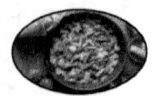

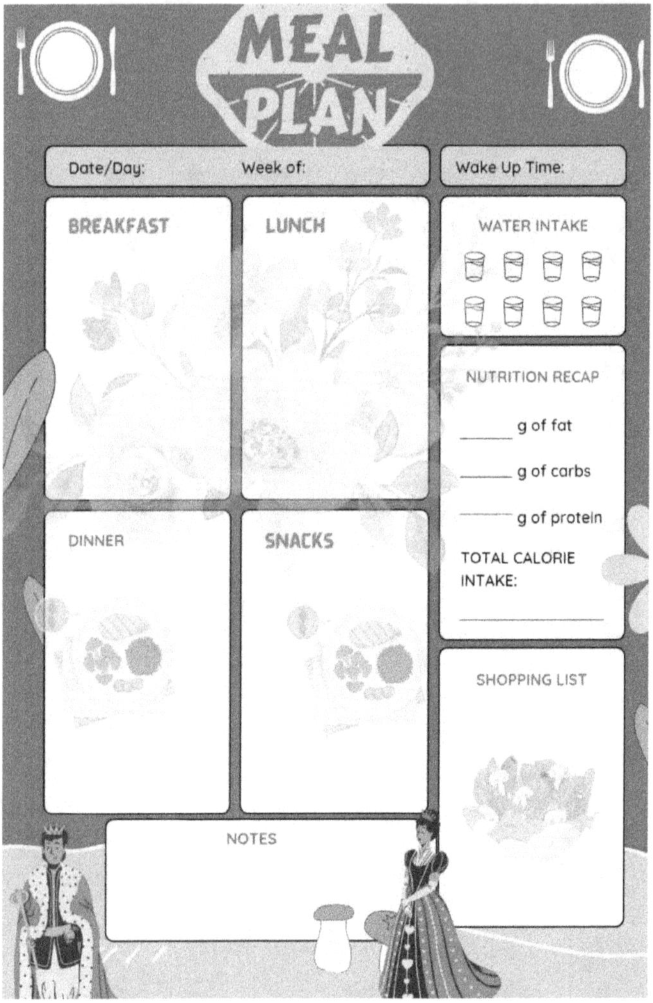

MEAL PLAN

| Date/Day: | Week of: | Wake Up Time: |

BREAKFAST

LUNCH

WATER INTAKE

NUTRITION RECAP

_____ g of fat

_____ g of carbs

_____ g of protein

TOTAL CALORIE INTAKE:

_____

DINNER

SNACKS

SHOPPING LIST

NOTES

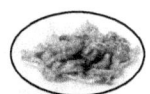
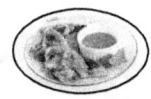
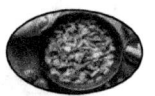

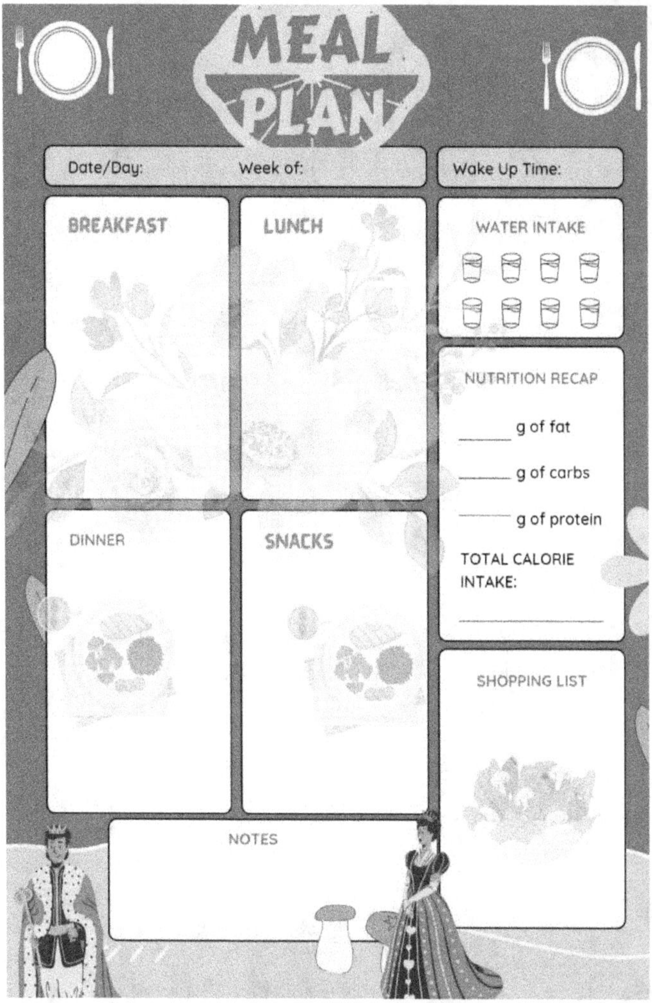

MEAL PLAN

Date/Day:	Week of:	Wake Up Time:

BREAKFAST

LUNCH

WATER INTAKE

NUTRITION RECAP

_____ g of fat

_____ g of carbs

_____ g of protein

TOTAL CALORIE INTAKE:

_____

DINNER

SNACKS

SHOPPING LIST

NOTES

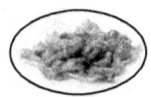 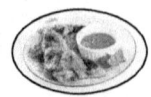 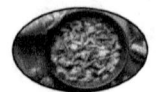

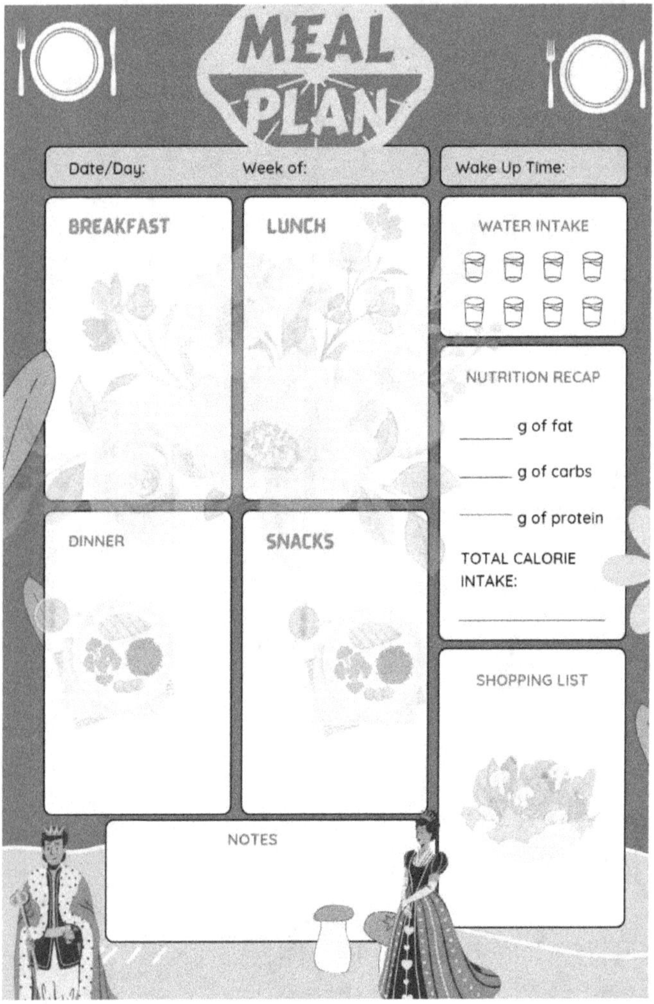

MEAL PLAN

| Date/Day: | Week of: | Wake Up Time: |

BREAKFAST

LUNCH

WATER INTAKE

NUTRITION RECAP

_____ g of fat

_____ g of carbs

_____ g of protein

TOTAL CALORIE INTAKE:

_____

DINNER

SNACKS

SHOPPING LIST

NOTES

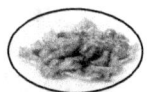 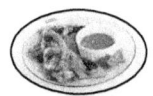 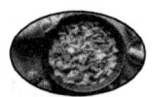

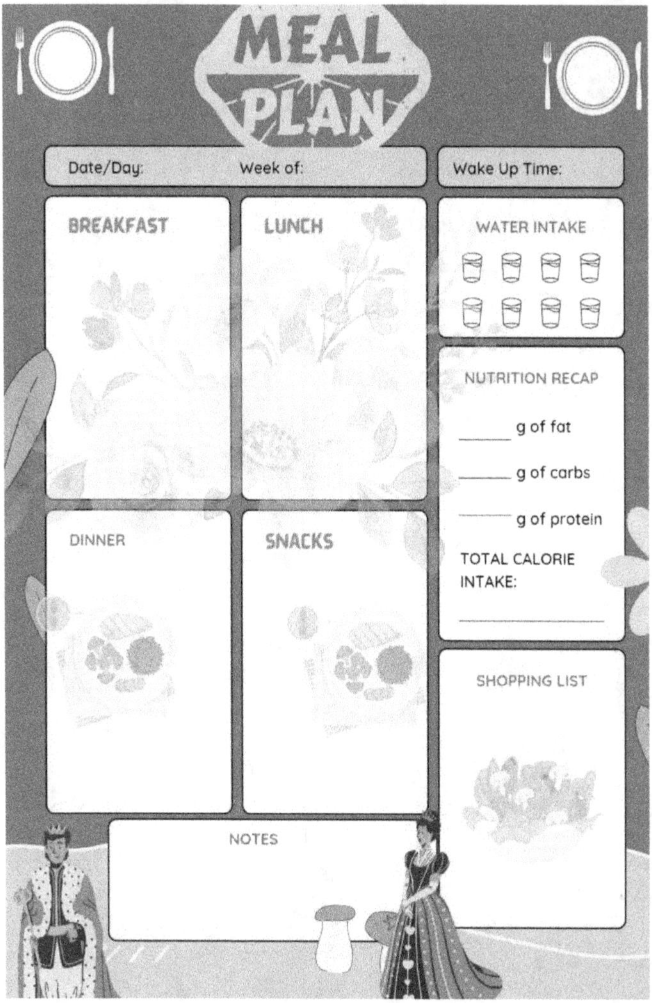

MEAL PLAN

| Date/Day: | Week of: | Wake Up Time: |

BREAKFAST

LUNCH

WATER INTAKE

NUTRITION RECAP

_____ g of fat

_____ g of carbs

_____ g of protein

TOTAL CALORIE INTAKE:

_____

DINNER

SNACKS

SHOPPING LIST

NOTES

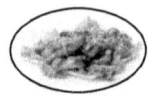 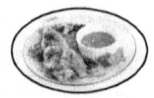 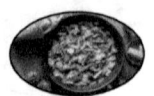

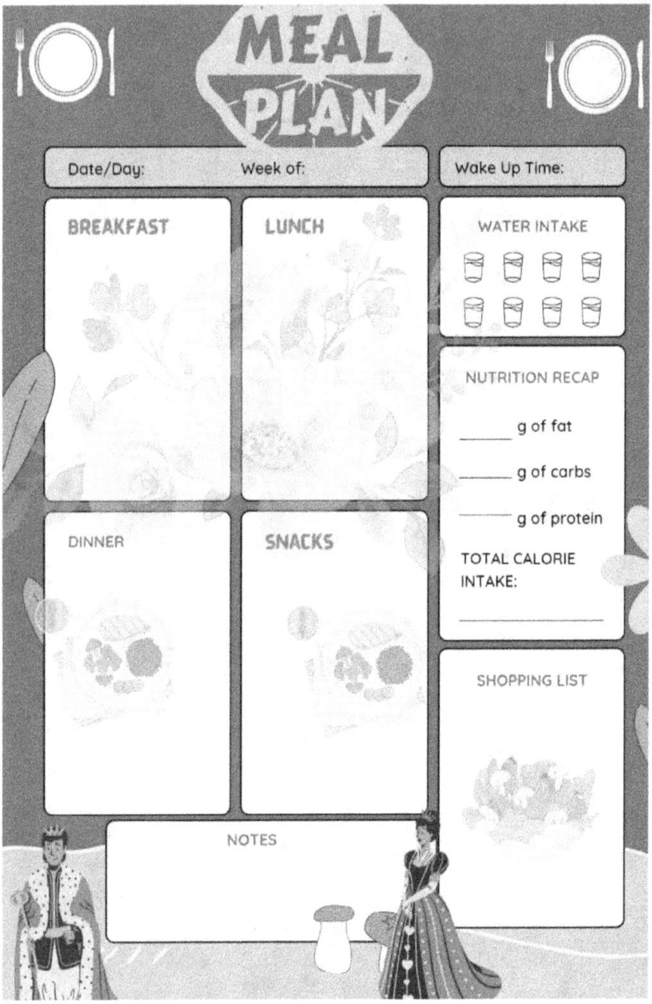

MEAL PLAN

Date/Day: | Week of: | Wake Up Time:

BREAKFAST

LUNCH

WATER INTAKE

NUTRITION RECAP

_____ g of fat

_____ g of carbs

_____ g of protein

TOTAL CALORIE INTAKE:

_____

DINNER

SNACKS

SHOPPING LIST

NOTES

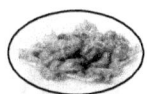 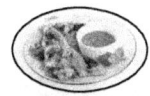 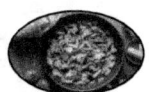

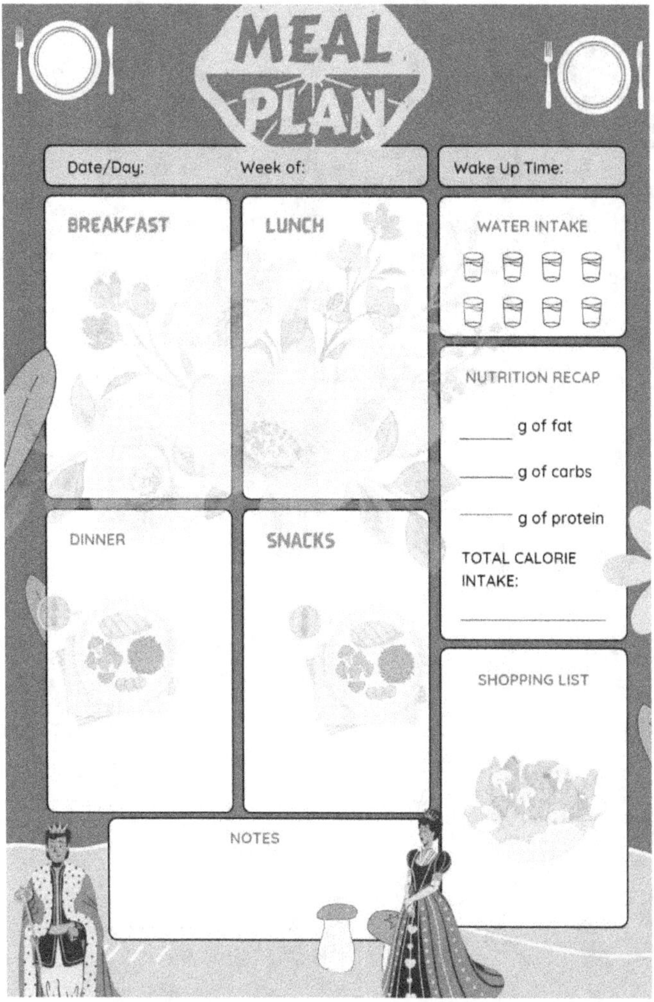

MEAL PLAN

Date/Day:	Week of:	Wake Up Time:

BREAKFAST

LUNCH

WATER INTAKE

NUTRITION RECAP

_____ g of fat

_____ g of carbs

_____ g of protein

TOTAL CALORIE INTAKE:

_____

DINNER

SNACKS

SHOPPING LIST

NOTES

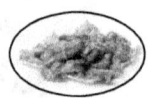 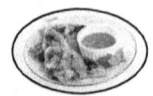 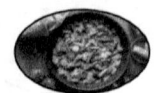

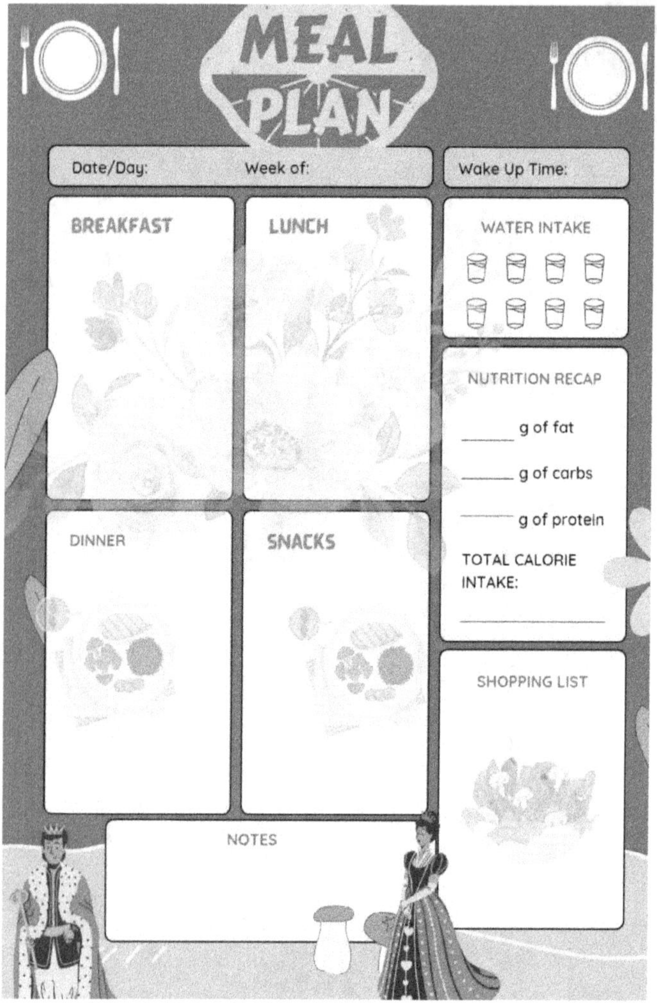

MEAL PLAN

| Date/Day: | Week of: | Wake Up Time: |

BREAKFAST

LUNCH

WATER INTAKE

NUTRITION RECAP

_____ g of fat

_____ g of carbs

_____ g of protein

TOTAL CALORIE INTAKE:

_____

DINNER

SNACKS

SHOPPING LIST

NOTES

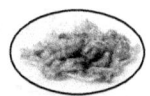
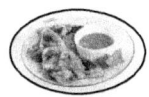
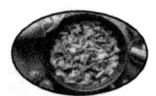

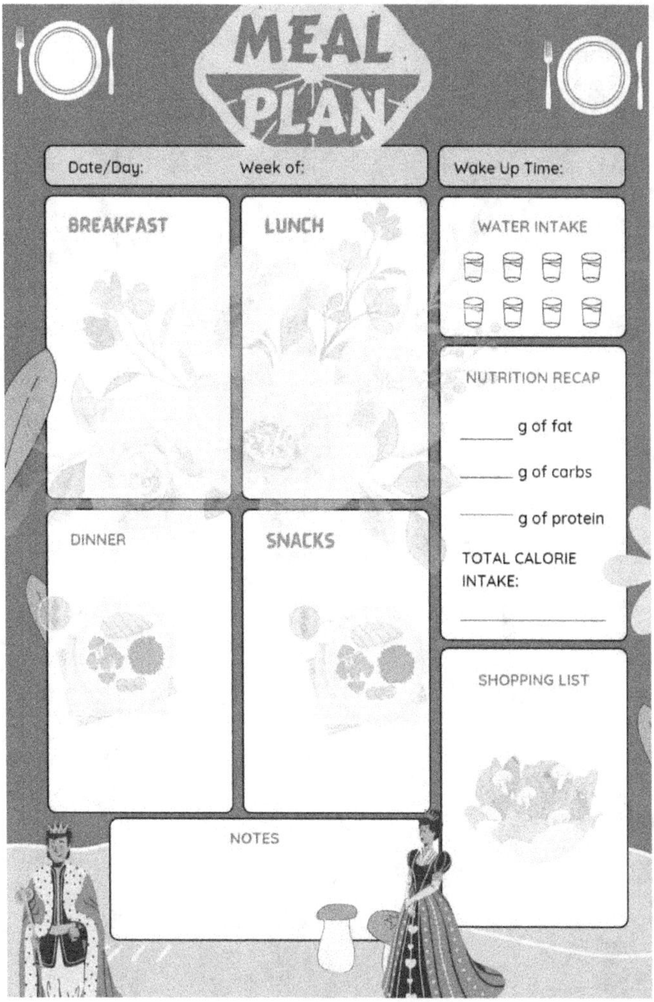

MEAL PLAN

| Date/Day: | Week of: | Wake Up Time: |

BREAKFAST

LUNCH

WATER INTAKE

NUTRITION RECAP

_____ g of fat

_____ g of carbs

_____ g of protein

TOTAL CALORIE INTAKE:

_____

DINNER

SNACKS

SHOPPING LIST

NOTES

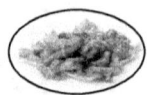
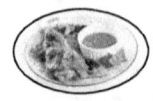
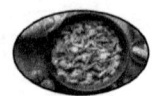

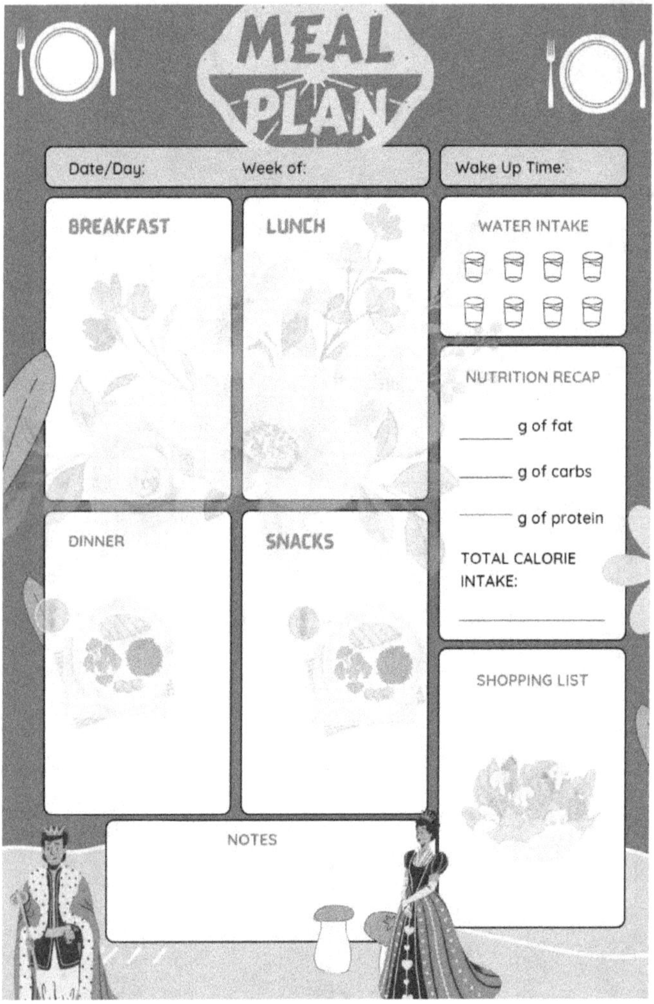

MEAL PLAN

| Date/Day: | Week of: | Wake Up Time: |

BREAKFAST

LUNCH

WATER INTAKE

NUTRITION RECAP

_____ g of fat

_____ g of carbs

_____ g of protein

TOTAL CALORIE INTAKE:
_____

DINNER

SNACKS

SHOPPING LIST

NOTES

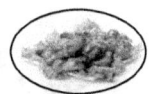
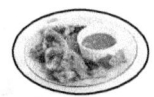
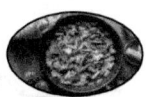

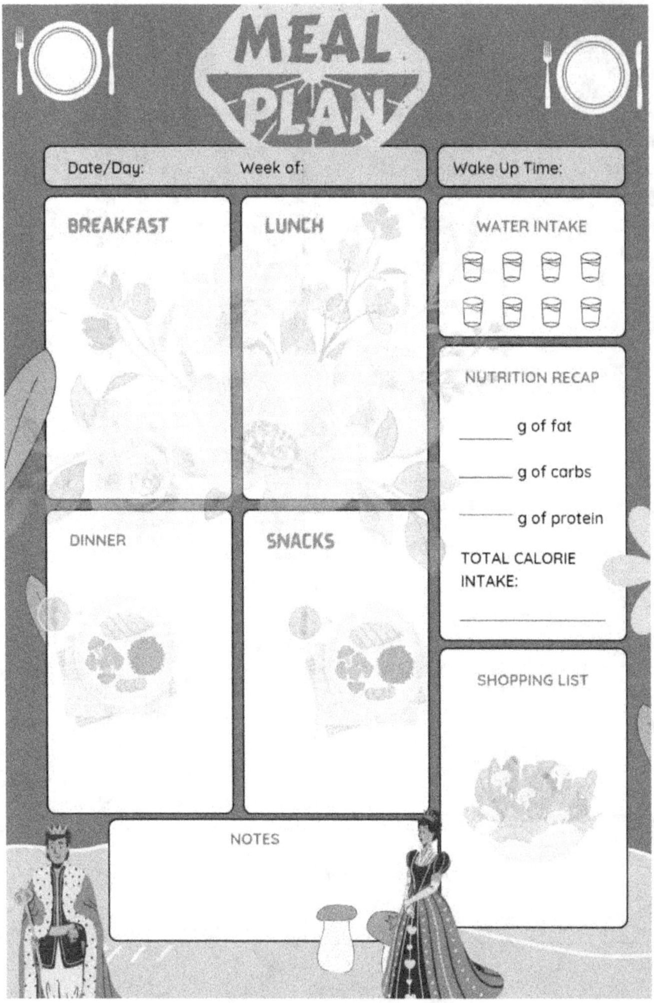

MEAL PLAN

Date/Day:	Week of:	Wake Up Time:

BREAKFAST

LUNCH

WATER INTAKE

NUTRITION RECAP

_____ g of fat

_____ g of carbs

_____ g of protein

TOTAL CALORIE INTAKE:

_____

DINNER

SNACKS

SHOPPING LIST

NOTES

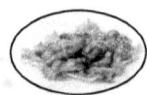 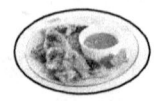 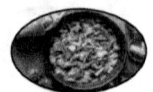

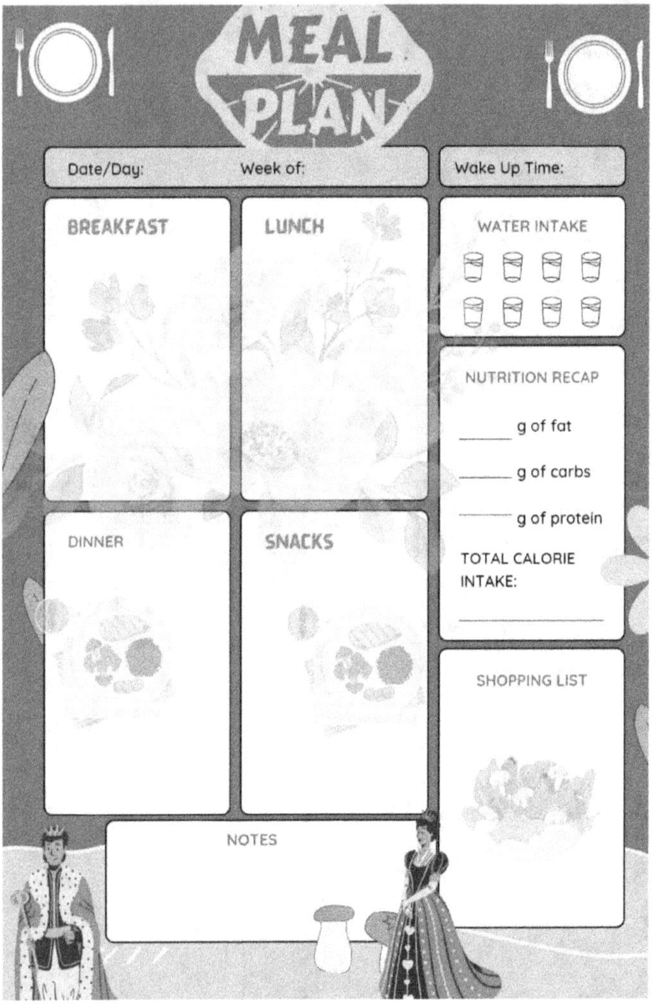

MEAL PLAN

Date/Day:	Week of:	Wake Up Time:

BREAKFAST

LUNCH

WATER INTAKE

NUTRITION RECAP

_____ g of fat

_____ g of carbs

_____ g of protein

TOTAL CALORIE INTAKE:
_____

DINNER

SNACKS

SHOPPING LIST

NOTES

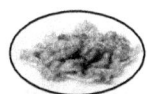 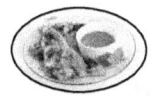 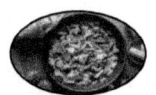

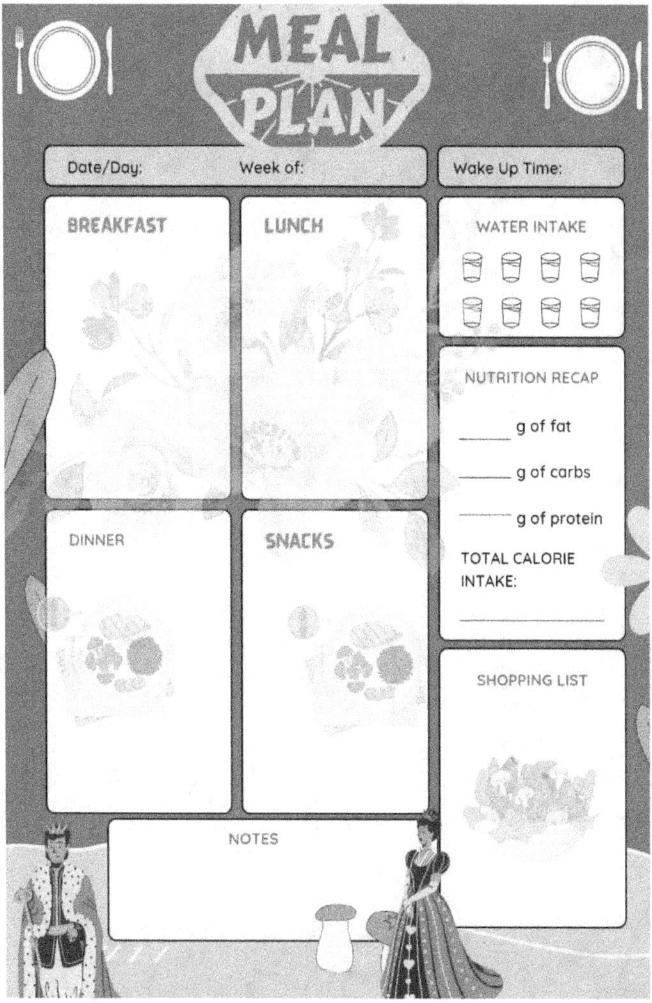

MEAL PLAN

| Date/Day: | Week of: | Wake Up Time: |

BREAKFAST

LUNCH

WATER INTAKE

NUTRITION RECAP

_____ g of fat

_____ g of carbs

_____ g of protein

TOTAL CALORIE INTAKE:

_____

DINNER

SNACKS

SHOPPING LIST

NOTES

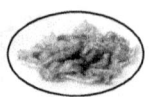 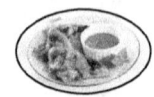 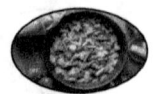

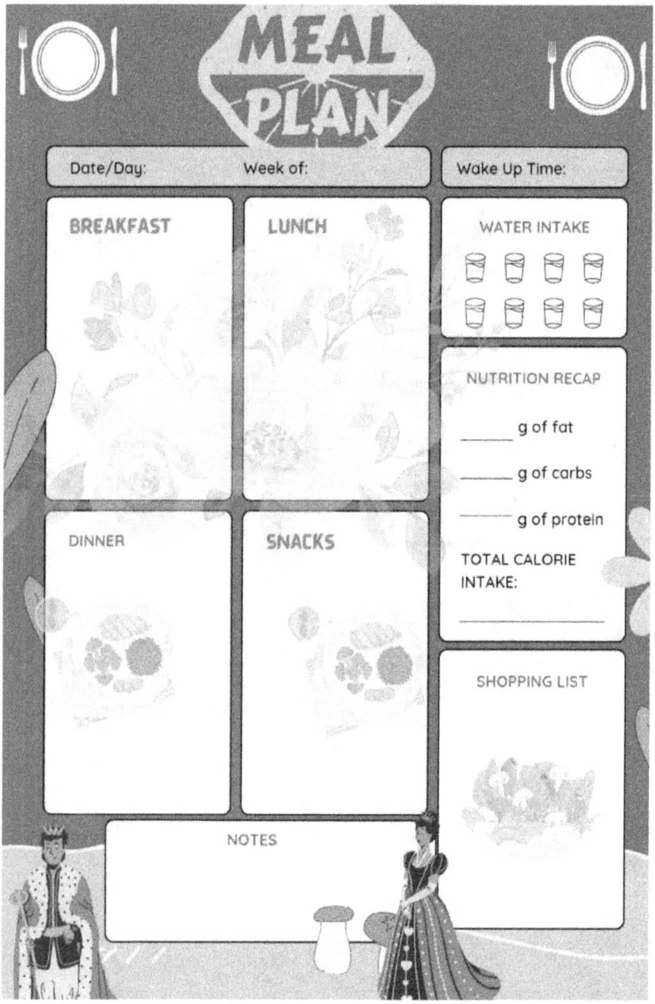

MEAL PLAN

| Date/Day: | Week of: | Wake Up Time: |

BREAKFAST

LUNCH

WATER INTAKE

NUTRITION RECAP

_____ g of fat

_____ g of carbs

_____ g of protein

TOTAL CALORIE INTAKE:

_____

DINNER

SNACKS

SHOPPING LIST

NOTES

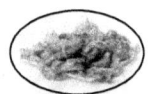 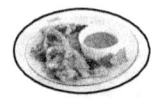 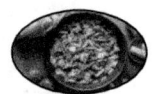

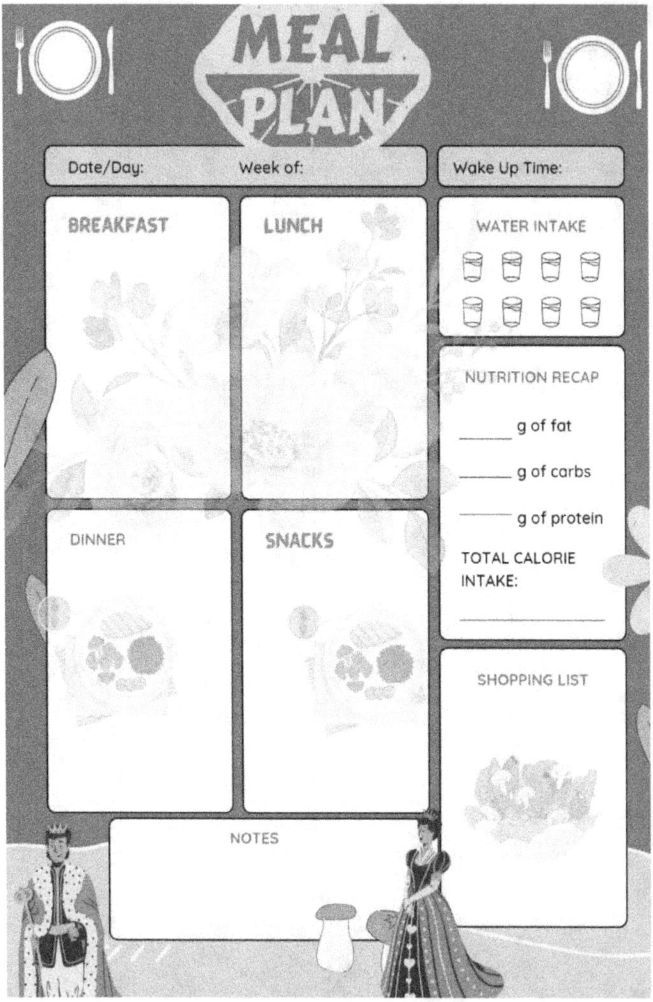

MEAL PLAN

Date/Day:	Week of:	Wake Up Time:

BREAKFAST

LUNCH

WATER INTAKE

NUTRITION RECAP

_____ g of fat

_____ g of carbs

_____ g of protein

TOTAL CALORIE INTAKE:

_____

DINNER

SNACKS

SHOPPING LIST

NOTES

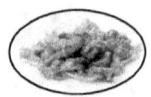 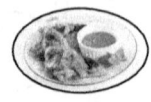 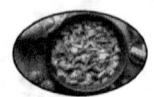

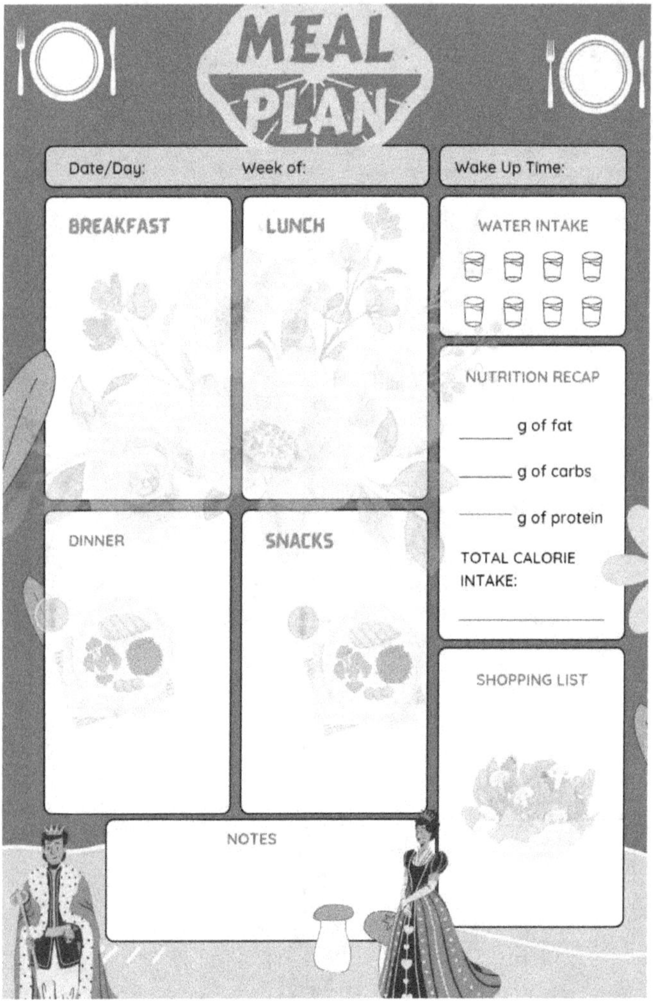

MEAL PLAN

Date/Day: **Week of:**   **Wake Up Time:**

BREAKFAST

LUNCH

WATER INTAKE

NUTRITION RECAP

_____ g of fat

_____ g of carbs

_____ g of protein

TOTAL CALORIE INTAKE:
_____

DINNER

SNACKS

SHOPPING LIST

NOTES

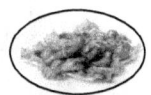
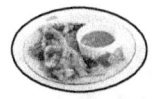
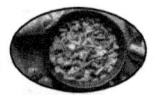

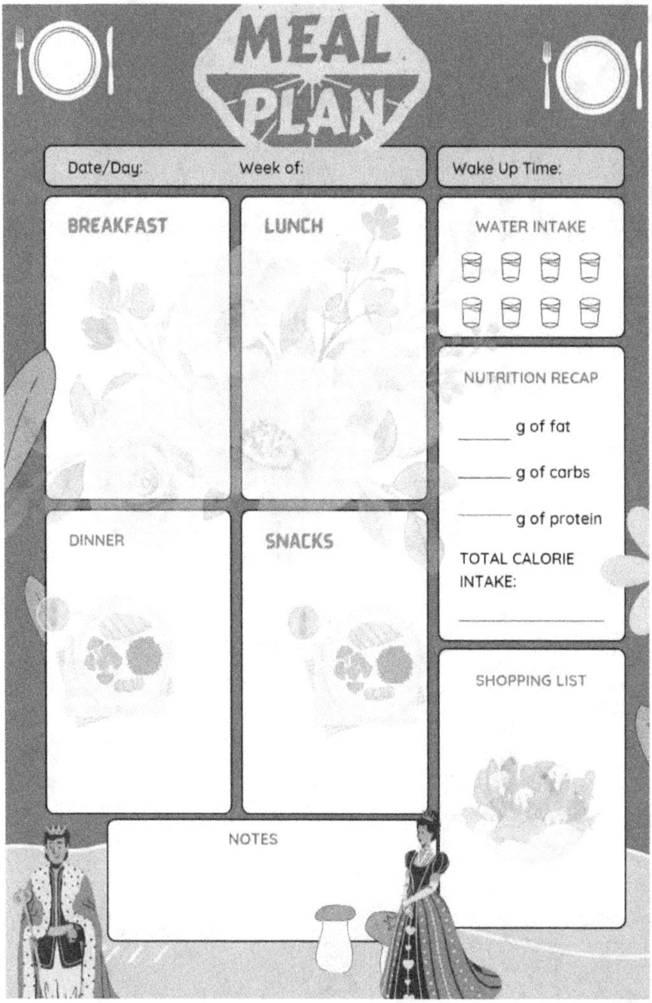

MEAL PLAN

Date/Day:	Week of:	Wake Up Time:

BREAKFAST

LUNCH

WATER INTAKE

NUTRITION RECAP

_____ g of fat

_____ g of carbs

_____ g of protein

TOTAL CALORIE INTAKE:

_____

DINNER

SNACKS

SHOPPING LIST

NOTES

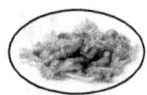 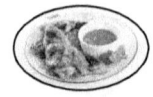 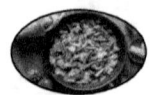

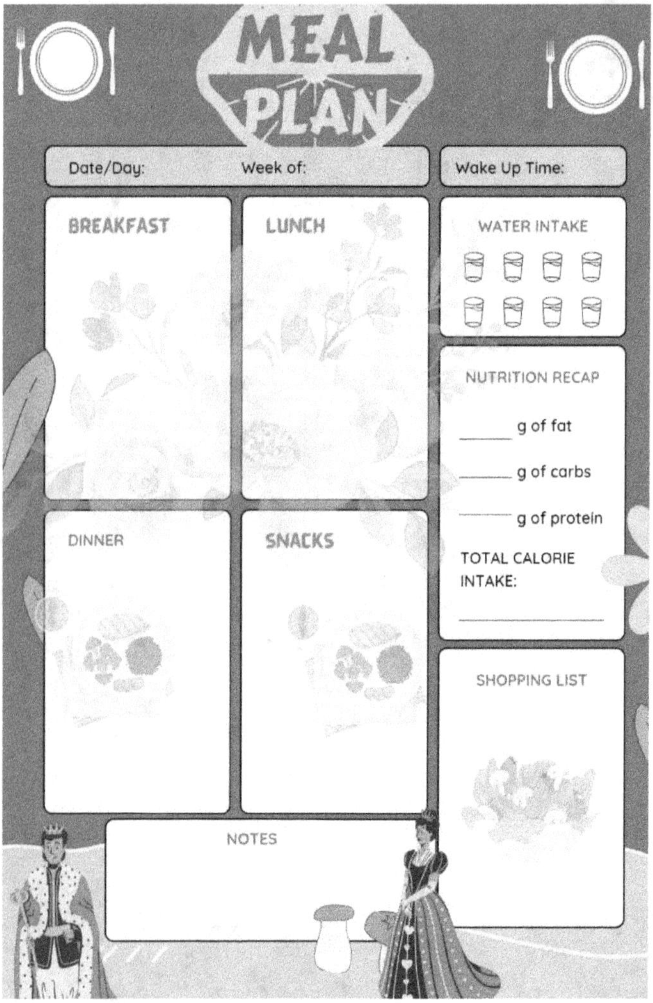

MEAL PLAN

Date/Day:	Week of:	Wake Up Time:

BREAKFAST

LUNCH

WATER INTAKE

NUTRITION RECAP

_____ g of fat

_____ g of carbs

_____ g of protein

TOTAL CALORIE INTAKE:

_____

DINNER

SNACKS

SHOPPING LIST

NOTES

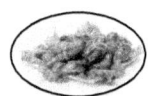 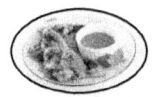 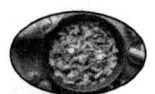

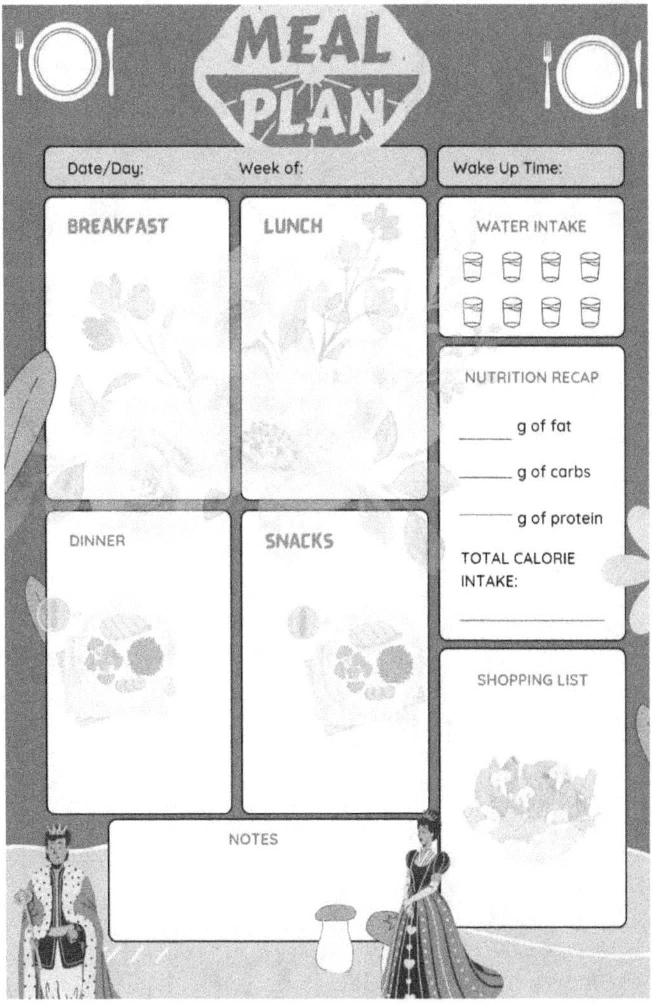

MEAL PLAN

| Date/Day: | Week of: | Wake Up Time: |

BREAKFAST

LUNCH

WATER INTAKE

NUTRITION RECAP

_____ g of fat

_____ g of carbs

_____ g of protein

TOTAL CALORIE INTAKE:

_____

DINNER

SNACKS

SHOPPING LIST

NOTES